30 Chic Days at Home
Vol. 2

*Creating a serene spa-like
ambience in your home for
soothing peace and relaxation*

FIONA FERRIS

ISBN: 9798862722628

Contents

Introduction 1

Day 1 - *Make your bed* 3

Day 2 - *Calm your senses with music* 6

Day 3 - *Create exquisite order in a spot in your home* 9

Day 4 - *Apply your makeup in a relaxed fashion.* 12

Day 5 - *Make yourself a spa snack* 15

Day 6 - *Curate your own lady basket* 18

Day 7 - *Infuse your home with fragrance* 21

Day 8 - *Dim the lights* 24

Day 9 - *Choose from your spa drink menu* 27

Day 10 - *Increase the beauty that surrounds you* 30

Day 11 - *Go on a walk outdoors* 33

Day 12 - *Create a 'contemplation corner'* 36

Day 13 - *Uplift yourself with happy journalling* .. 39

Day 14 - *Introduce pampering spa touches* 43

Day 15 - *Be in a soft, hushed atmosphere* 46

Day 16 - *Nourish yourself three times a day* 49

Day 17 - *Partake in boudoir time* 52

Day 18 - *Browse your style files* 55

Day 19 - *Indulge yourself every day* 58

Day 20 - *Love herbal tea* 61

Day 21 - *Take time to dream* 64

Day 22 - *Decrease your to-do list* 67

Day 23 - *Be slow* 70

Day 24 - *Create a sense of calm in your home* 73

Day 25 - *Always be streamlining* 76

Day 26 - *Practice reflexology daily* 79

Day 27 - *Find five minutes for stretching* 82

Day 28 - *Connect with girlfriends* 85

Day 29 - *Develop morning and evening rituals* .. 88

Day 30 - *Create your own spa day* 92

21 Ways to make your home a calm haven 96

To finish 103

About the author 105

Other books by Fiona Ferris 107

Introduction

In July of this year, I started a series on my blog 'How to be Chic' called *Serene Spa July*, where I wrote about many small ways you can bring about the restful feeling of being at a spa, but at home. To embody the spa ambience for yourself and your own wellbeing. You know, that floaty spacious feeling you get from walking into, or even just viewing a photo of, a high-end spa. But we're doing it for zero dollars, ourselves.

This book is a refined and expanded version of the blog series, edited and polished into a cute book to inspire you to create a luxurious spa-like existence for yourself in your everyday life. It is quick to read, and the print version is adorable, perfect for sliding into your bag for a refreshing few minutes when you have to wait somewhere.

Maybe you have some good habits down pat: daily walks, drinking water, and keeping your food nutritious for the most part, plus serving yourself portion sizes that are not too big.

And perhaps there are other areas you would like to improve upon. You've decided that you'd like to add in some more stretching, downtime with a book, and in general rest and recuperation.

Many of us are always on the go-go-go which is quite ironic considering we love to dream of a calm, peaceful and serene life. I think we dream of it *because* we're always on the go! It's for us to hear and absorb!

As you read through this book, ask yourself what one or two things you would love to add in for yourself as a focus through the thirty days. Note them down or incorporate them straight away.

My wish is that you will receive loads of value and fun inspiration from this book. I really hope you enjoy it!

With good wishes from beautiful Hawke's Bay, New Zealand,

Fiona

Day 1 -
Make your bed

Your first tip is to *make your bed as early in the day as possible*. As I write this it is just before 7.30am, and I have already made my bed. I know, I am impressed too! I cannot say that every day but in this series of *30 Chic Days at Home* I certainly will be. And then it will be a good habit, yay!

Our goal for the month is to bring about the spa-like feeling of peace and relaxation into our lives, so a neatly made bed will be happening early every day.

There are so many benefits!

- You will receive a feeling of accomplishment
- Your bedroom will look neater and tidier in only five minutes
- Your day will be started off right
- You will be encouraged to keep your bedroom

tidier than if your bed was unmade
- You've already got one job ticked off
- You get to enjoy the serene vista for longer than if you made your bed later in the day
- A neat bedroom will put you in a better mood
- It will also boost your productivity (an object in motion stays in motion!)
- You will feel a sense of calm
- And your sleep will be improved as you climb into a neatly made bed tonight

I even read a study that said people who make their bed each day earn more than those who don't. I can't see how this would come about, but why take a chance on your financial future?

You may already be an early bed maker so good on you. But do you have pets?

Unfortunately my little dogs Daphne and Chloe *love* to mess the bed up for me. Chloe jumps over behind the decorative pillow in the middle *all the time*, then flips around knocking all the pillows over.

If you don't have pets, you really don't know the 'fun' you are missing out on... Still, I straighten up the pillows when necessary, it only takes a second.

My favourite reasons for making my bed early in the day are that I feel productive, and also that my room is pleasing to view multiple times a day since I work from home. But even for those of us who go into an office every day, how much nicer would it be to come home from a long day at work to a neatly made bed than otherwise?

30 Chic Days at Home inspired action:

Have you made your bed yet today? If not, quickly do it and feel happy with your achievement!

Day 2 -

Calm your senses with music

When I am at home, and even when I'm out (I leave it on for the doggies when they can't come with me), I have soft music playing in the central hallway of our home. It's one of my favourite kinds of self-care and the first thing I do in the morning is switch on my music.

I love the way it filters into my office and that I can hear it as I move around the house but it's never too loud.

I switch between actual flutey spa music, background jazz, and anything that is soft and instrumental. You can search for 'background music', 'study music' or 'spa music' on YouTube, and I have a playlist on Spotify called 'Dior Relaxing Music' that I sometimes play too.

It is a recreation of a CD I was given when I worked at Dior in their head office almost twenty years ago, and it was played while ladies had a 'Silver Method' facial with one of the Dior consultants. I have just about worn my CD out and thankfully was able to save it forever on Spotify!

I used to play it before I went to sleep, but nowadays I play it during the day. It is guaranteed to relax me instantly. (You can listen to it too by searching for 'Dior Relaxing Music' on Spotify and you'll find it under my name 'Fiona Ferris').

You might prefer calming classical music or another type altogether, but if you have a little music setup, you can play soft music all day every day. I don't want to tie my phone up, so I use our very, very old iPod which has all my music loaded onto it and it sits in our very, very old iPod dock. But it's perfect for what I want!

Maybe there is something you can repurpose too. Perhaps you have a CD player to play relaxing music on.

The best thing about streaming YouTube, Spotify or similar though is that you never have to change the disc. And you can play many different songs on 'shuffle' so you never tire of the same CD.

The main thing to consider is that this music does not have a singer – it's purely instrumental in whatever genre is your favourite. Then you can easily study, work, or chat with it on in the background and it doesn't interfere with your thoughts. It just relaxes and calms you very gently and very easily.

It's wonderful!

30 Chic Days at Home inspired action:

Research different kinds of relaxing music and choose your preference to play as a gentle background when you are at home or work.

Day 3 -
Create exquisite order in a spot in your home

Having a tidy environment is a key ingredient in a relaxed and harmonious home, but you don't have to plan for a huge cleanout to be able to benefit. Even just one small area tidied up will help you feel amazing.

Yesterday I cleaned out and reorganized my side of the bathroom cupboard, plus the drawer I keep my perfumes in. I have a lot of perfume! But I enjoy it and wear it every day, plus I like to have variety. I would love to be someone who has a signature fragrance but I would get so bored!

I took everything out, wiped the drawer and cupboard shelves clean, then put things back. I didn't put as much back though. I threw out three products that I know I will never use, and it was such a feeling of relief.

In total the cost would be less than $10 and yet I'd had those items hanging around for a long time feeling bad that I didn't want to use them! I am not usually wasteful *at all* and use everything up that I've ever bought one way or another, but yesterday I thought 'I'm better than that'. Some of us think about things more than other people and it can keep us feeling stuck!

I also rehomed a few backup items to a different area, into a container that I can 'shop' from when I run out, such as shampoo and body wash. I don't need to cram all backups into my small bathroom cupboard.

And I did a cool thing that is going to be so useful. I had three extra turntables from my pantry, and put those in the cleaned out bathroom cupboard. It is so luxurious to be able to see all my body lotions and body sprays by twirling them around. I like to choose different scents to wear each day, so now nothing gets hidden at the back!

I know there are tons of little areas like this all over my home, and I'm sure you will have quite a few as well. The good news is that it can take as little as 15-30 minutes to straighten up a space, and you will receive many times that amount of good feeling back for your effort.

30 Chic Days at Home inspired action:

Find one small area that is bothering you, and create beautiful order in that space. It might even be one shelf. Don't overwhelm yourself. But do try and do it as fast as you can so it doesn't become a big ordeal, and then bask in the glow of that neatened space.

Day 4 -

Apply your makeup in a relaxed fashion

I love how beauticians, aestheticians and makeup counter salesladies are always beautifully made up. Their *maquillage* is impeccable with a poreless complexion, richly pigmented lipstick, and enviable eye makeup. How do they do it so well?

Practice, my friend.

I still practice my eye makeup each day. Even after all these years of doing it I know I still need to push myself out of my comfort zone and try new things. Of course on busy days I'll do it quickly, but even if I have five or ten extra minutes it's a chance to go a little bolder in the eye area.

And when you don't have as much time, a brighter lipstick than usual is your best bet. I always admire a bold lip on a lady and often observe how it brightens her whole face up.

I know we all prefer differing amounts of makeup. Personally I believe that any face can be improved with even a little. Plus it's a creative way to spend ten minutes with an enjoyable audiobook or listenable YouTube video. Or, if you want to try a new look, follow along a makeup tutorial video on YouTube. I have picked up so many little tricks from watching a few.

You don't have to buy expensive makeup either. I have mixed in drugstore brands with the occasional pricier item for a long time. Even inexpensive foundations are much better than they used to be.

The only area where I see a difference is with eyeshadows. The less expensive palettes don't seem to have much oomph to their colour, whereas a higher-end eyeshadow palette seems to be finer and have more pigment. Try them on your hand before buying to make sure you are actually getting some colour for your money!

30 Chic Days at Home inspired action:

Clean out your makeup collection and commit to using what you own. If anything is too old, throw it out. Mascaras should be replaced regularly, whereas a palette such as eyeshadow or blush, if it looks and smells good you should be fine. And if you notice your lipstick that you've had for a while no longer smells so fresh, get rid of that too. It's better to use fewer items and replace them regularly.

For example, I only have one mascara at a time now, and use it every day. At around the 3-4 month mark it starts to feel a little dry, and that's when I replace it. It's healthier for your eyes to do it this way rather than have a collection of mascaras that you use occasionally and keep for years.

You will be inspired to use your makeup more with a streamlined collection. And while you're at it, clean up the cases of the items you are keeping. A clean lint-free cloth and a bottle of your least favourite perfume will do this beautifully.

Day 5 -
Make yourself a spa snack

Many years ago, my brother won a couples massage at a five-star hotel. Because he was single at the time he took me as his plus-one. Thank goodness we were in separate rooms is all I can say! It was a blissful experience and such a nice treat.

Afterwards we lay on loungers in white fluffy robes while a light snack was served to us: herbal tea, dried apricots, raw almonds, and dates which felt so elegant and were delicious to nibble on. Plus, nutritious!

It made me think how good it would be to have a mini-menu of healthy snacks at home too. Any of us can do this for ourselves easily and feel like we are lying on those loungers relaxing. Here are my favourite ideas for a spa snack:

- As above, dried fruits and raw nuts in a small dish.
- Fresh fruit washed, sliced, and displayed nicely.
- A small portion of unsweetened Greek yoghurt with apple chopped into it. This snack tides me over until dinnertime if I get hungry in the afternoon.
- Crudités and a little hummus.
- Chia seed pudding with fresh fruit and nut butter.

You will find that not only do these types of snacks satisfy you sooner than if you ate something more refined like a chocolate bar, but that you will feel better afterwards. Your blood sugar won't spike and crash, and you will also feel good from the nutrients.

If you think it is boring to 'eat healthy' as I used to, reframe that same food to be a 'spa snack' and plate it prettily. You will find it much more appealing.

And it doesn't have to just be about replacing unhealthy snacks with healthy alternatives either. Creating a spa menu for any of your meals could bring about deliciously nutritious results.

The first thought that comes to mind for me is that a meal at a health spa would have additional ingredients such as fresh herbs, microgreens, and 'good fat' foods like avocado and olive oil. I eat some of these things, but not all the time. However if I was to make my home into a health spa for a week, I'd be sure to add extra touches to all my meals.

It's just a different way of looking at how we eat and asking ourselves, 'How can I make this meal as healthy, delicious, and appealing as possible?' rather than 'What would taste good right now?' which sometimes often leads to less healthful choices. This is definitely true for me!

30 Chic Days at Home inspired action:

Set yourself up at home so you can enjoy a spa snack any time you feel like it. Dried fruit and raw nuts keep well in the pantry, and fruit stays crisp in the fridge. (But if you don't use your raw nuts very quickly, they might be better stored in the fridge too.)

And think about what extra touches you can add to meals in order to increase their taste, beauty and nutrient content.

Day 6 -

Curate your own lady basket

A while back my husband Paul noticed how much I carry around with me – a book, my journal, phone, pen, water bottle etc. From my desk to the living room, to beside our bed were the three main spots. At any one time I could be transporting a large number of items. I would carry a teetering pile or else had to do two trips!

He suggested that I needed a basket to carry everything in (half-joking, half-not), and this is how 'the lady basket' was born. I thought it was such an excellent idea and repurposed a flat woven cane basket with a handle at each end. It does the job perfectly.

Isn't the name just so cute? I mean, who wouldn't love to have their own lady basket? And, of course, it's very handy too. You won't have items lying around. Your desk or side table will look neater because all your items are corralled into one container. Plus, all you have to do is pick it up and take it with you.

You can put whatever items in your lady basket that are useful to you. But make sure to clean it out often. You don't want a big heavy lady basket with tons of stuff in it. Keep it to only the items you use often.

In my lady basket are:

- My phone
- iPad
- Kindle
- Reading glasses
- A notepad
- AirPods
- Journal
- Pen
- And my current book or magazine that I'm reading

If you think this is the kind of thing you need, take a look around and see if you already own a suitable container. I'm always a fan of using what I have as a first choice, both for not wasting money, and also the clutter factor.

This is an 'at home' lady basket, but you could also do something similar in the trunk of your car, with a tote housing items such as a bottle of water, your umbrella or rain jacket, and some shopping bags. These things are usually in your car of course, but actually putting them into a container to keep them neat is next level organized. It's so satisfying!

30 Chic Days at Home inspired action:

Curate *your* own lady basket. And then, there is the fun of working out what you want in it. You can be inspired by mine, and also add any extras that you would find useful such as tissues, your current needlecraft project, handcream, mints in a tin... there really is an endless array of items that may be useful.

Day 7 -
Infuse your home with fragrance

Creating a bespoke fragrance for your home is something that is often forgotten, but makes a huge difference to your sense of peace and wellbeing. Have you ever walked into a hotel lobby that has a beautiful white tea fragrance piped through? Or entered a store with an exquisitely scented candle burning? Fragrance adds an extra dimension of pleasure and luxury'; it is a facet we cannot see but definitely take in.

There are a few different ways in which to create a beautiful fragrance in your home. Some of my favourites include:

- Lighting scented candles
- Using wax melts
- Diffusing essential oils
- Burning incense

- Perfumed room spray
- Automatic fragrance misters

I love to light a candle in the hall so it wafts throughout the whole house. I also have an essential oil diffuser in my office which smells beautiful.

Favourite 'recipes' for my diffuser (usually three drops of each essential oil) include:

Orange, geranium, lavender
Lemon, mandarin, peppermint
Lavender, lime, orange

I am a fan of citrus essential oils, and lighter fragrances overall, but in the holiday season it is fun to diffuse a seasonal essential oil with ingredients such as clove and cinnamon.

If you gather together essential oils that appeal to your nose, you can create your own blends by putting two or three together in your diffuser.

There are other ways to make your home smell wonderful too:

- Using naturally scented or fine fragrance cleaning and laundry products.
- Throwing the windows open each day even if only for a short while.
- Keeping dusting, vacuuming, and bedding

changes up-to-date. Clean smells clean!

- Baking or cooking a cozy meal.
- Putting on a pot of coffee.

You may be a 'fresh air' person who doesn't like a lot of fragrance, which means a clean home, unscented home care products, open windows, and fresh flowers.

A room that is decluttered and with the right amount of furniture and possessions in it goes a long way too. If a home is overly full and cannot be cleaned effectively, there may be an underlying scent of must.

Keeping this in mind helps me always be moving along items that I haven't used in a long time. I want to live in a clean, fresh-smelling home, not a dusty museum!

30 Chic Days at Home inspired action:

Consider your preference when it comes to the scent of your home. Do you prefer bakery fragranced candles or fresh-smelling essential oils? Could you open your windows right now? Wash the dog blankets more often? Spring clean a room?

Day 8 -
Dim the lights

The right lighting makes a huge difference to the look and feel of your home, and that's why I love having different options such as ceiling lights, wall lights and lamps. During the day when I'm productive writing books at my desk and moving around the house doing chores, I have the lights on bright in my office, and in the rooms I am using such as the kitchen.

In other rooms like our dark-painted living room which has a moody deep vibe, I keep table lamps on all day. I love the look and cozy feel when I pass through that room, no matter the season.

And after dinner it is soothing to switch off overhead lights and keep only the lamps on. Doing this means our minds are calmed and we can begin to wind down for sleep time.

Dimmer switches on lights are great for this too. Whenever we've had any electrical work done, I switch out that room's light switch for a dimmer. Slowly I am making my way around the house!

And even if you don't want to go to the expense of having an electrician come around, there are many bulb options these days including smart bulbs that you can dim or change colour from an app on your phone. You will be amazed if you haven't been into a lighting store lately. The new LED bulbs are more expensive, but it's nice not to have to change them as often. Plus they are cheaper to run, and don't heat up like old-fashioned bulbs either. This can be better for the fittings they are in, so the higher up-front cost is somewhat reasonable when you take all this into account.

As with my dimmer switch makeovers, I buy the new-style bulbs as and when I need them so the cost is spread out. You can choose cool-tone bulbs for rooms that need to be brightly lit such as in the garage or laundry, and warm-tone bulbs for a softer look in living areas. There are even fancy designer bulbs that are as much a feature as the shade they are in. These bulbs can be pricey, but if they are a design detail might be worth it.

All of this corresponds nicely with being at a high-end spa. The moment you walk in it's hushed and softly lit and you feel like you have been offered an invitation into peace and calm.

We can make our home feel like that too by just tweaking the lighting around us!

30 Chic Days at Home inspired action:

Start with one room and see if there are any minor changes you can make to the lighting.

Something that I'd really love to do in the future is have wall sconces as reading lights by our bed instead of bedside lamps. There will be less clutter on our nightstands, and having a reading light by the bed will feel very five-star hotel!

Day 9 -

Choose from your spa drink menu

When you visit a spa or if you have ever watched a television series where the characters are at a spa, you will see that a simple yet delicious drink is often served. Perhaps it will be fruit-infused water, or sparkling water.

It's so simple to do this at home by slicing washed fruit into water and storing it in the fridge. Lemons and other citrus, fresh berries, and even slices of cucumber are all delicious. Use what is in season and least expensive, or even better, what you have growing at home. F R E E is always preferable, and freshest too!

We have the best little lime tree in our yard which is *so* prolific. I freeze washed quarters and use them for ice cubes in my cold drinks, and also in my smoothies. And I've squeezed them and made ice cubes from them too. Imagine dropping a lime juice

ice cube into your sparkling water along with a few slices of citrus, how delicious!

And don't forget about herbs. They are lovely in water as well – a sprig of mint flavours water delicately, and looks wonderful.

I also enjoy steeping herbal tea bags in cold water to sip on throughout the day, as an alternative to plain water. Favourites of mine are mint tea, lemon-flavoured green tea, and specialty cold infusion fruit teas. I leave the tea bag in, except for the green tea bag which I take out after fifteen minutes.

And if you want to level up your spa drink game, you could stock your fridge with coconut water, aloe vera juice, kombucha, or green juice.

But for day-to-day sipping, infused waters are perfect. They are flavoursome as well as being hydrating and refreshing, and do not add calories into your diet. There are plenty of recipes online and you can create your own infusions. How about strawberry, lemon, and basil? Or watermelon and mint?

The key is to prepare your fruit- or tea-infused water the night before so it's had plenty of time to flavour and chill. I love to have my spa waters icy cold for sipping, especially in the summer, but I prefer room temperature water for my plain eight glasses a day.

It feels so lovely and special to sip on your spa water, and it's a nice touch to offer to guests as well.

30 Chic Days at Home inspired action:

Find flavours you enjoy and play around with 'recipes'. Make it a habit to keep a bottle or jug in the fridge and enjoy the delicious flavour – and hydration benefits – of making water more palatable.

Day 10 -

Increase the beauty that surrounds you

Even in the home you currently live in, and without going out and buying anything new, you can raise the level of beauty in your environment. It's amazing how even a few small touches can elevate the feeling of your home.

Creating beauty, and infusing your home with a sense of calm elegance is something you can do every day.

- Set a beautiful table for dinner (most of us have lovely dishes and napery that we rarely bring out)
- Tidy away surface clutter such as half-read magazines and newspapers. They can be stacked neatly if still in use.

- Bring elements of nature into a room with faux or fresh flowers, or a potted plant.
- Cluster small groups of ornaments or candles together rather than spreading them around. A home stager gave me this tip when she was photographing our last house for sale.
- Rotate décor items so they seem fresh in different areas or even different rooms. Art on the wall can be moved around too.

Something you can do today, is to take photos of the rooms in your house. Don't change anything before you do, and then look at them to see what stands out. There will be quick, obvious upgrades to sort out such as making your bed or clearing a tabletop.

And then look at the other details that catch your eye (not in a good way). I read that home magazine photographers tape lamp cords to a table leg if they are visible, as an example.

There are so many things we can do to increase the beauty in our home. I love to think of the term 'elegant lifestyle' or 'elegant living'. Keeping this phrase in mind inspires me to do even five minutes of tidying and beautifying.

30 Chic Days at Home inspired action:

Act as if you were an interior design expert brought in to do a makeover on this client's home. They have asked you to come in and see what changes can be done to make the space more attractive on a zero dollars budget. And, you're only being paid for a thirty minute consultation, so you'd better whizz around quickly!

Do a quick tidy up, look for tucked away treasures that can be used, and move things around. It's so fun to visit your home with fresh eyes and a new persona!

Day 11 -
Go on a walk outdoors

Whether you live in the city or country, and no matter if it's sunny or cold outside, take yourself for an outdoor walk. It doesn't have to be long, but at least go for a stroll to get some vitamin D, a few lungfuls of fresh air, and to look at the sights around you.

There is something that is so refreshing about being outside, even if you're in a built-up area. When we lived close to the city I used to love going for a glam walk. A glam walk combines exercise with window shopping. I'd wear nice clothes with sneakers, and exercise while I window-shopped. Big sunglasses were mandatory for this look!

Even with a lot of people around, I find it peaceful and relaxing to just stroll. And it's a great way to get your steps in without even noticing it too. As mentioned, the key is to wear nice sneakers with your outfit so that you're comfortable.

But mostly I would do my daily walks around the neighbourhood in the suburb we lived in. I wore exercise clothing for these walks – leggings and a tee-shirt.

I live in the countryside now, so I walk my doggies down the road, and we sometimes ramble through our paddock. The cows in there are always very curious and sometimes get a little playful! I normally keep the dogs away from them in case they get stood on. One time when it was cold both dogs had their hot-pink fleece jackets on and they were chased! Just like the 'red rag to a bull' saying, even though these were petite lady cows, not bulls.

And, if you don't have a dog, heed the advice to 'walk your dog every day, whether you have one or not'. I heard this saying ages ago and it's such a cute instruction. And sensible!

When I visit our small-town shops, it feels good to walk more too – I feel very European. Rather than move my car all over town, I park in one area and walk everywhere I need to go if I have the time and it's nice weather.

And whenever we visit the city and stay at a hotel right in town, I love being a tourist, dressing up and going for a walk around the city. As with my glam walks, I wear a nice outfit with trendy sneakers and stroll around, tourist-style.

Often on a trip you are sitting for long periods of time whether it's in the car or on an aeroplane. And then there are all the treat meals when you are on holiday, so it feels good to go for a refreshing, scenic walk each day!

30 Chic Days at Home inspired action:

See if you can go for an outdoor walk *today*. If it's freezing, rug up. If it's blazing, put your sunglasses on and find shade to walk in. Maybe you have a busy public park available to you with plenty of trees to cool you down. It feels good to go for a walk with people around; everyone looks so relaxed and happy!

Day 12 -

Create a 'contemplation corner'

When we lived in the city we used to stay at our favourite five-star hotel as our 'staycation' once or twice a year. In their spa area by the pool was a long room with comfortable seating and glossy magazines, and it was called the Contemplation Corner.

I borrowed their tranquil atmosphere and now enjoy creating contemplation corners in my own home. And you can too! It might involve turning a chair slightly so your view is out the window, and adding a temporarily-moved side table. Get yourself a vintage or current magazine or book, and a cold or hot drink and you are set for a little restorative solitude.

Alternatives include setting up a blanket under a tree outside. Or wrapping yourself snugly in a cozy rug on your sofa or bed for a while. You can even relax in your car if you are out, listening to an audiobook with a hot coffee. I love being in my car like this!

But my favourite is to be at home with a cup of tea and an old *Victoria* magazine. I choose an issue from my small collection and flip away for a little while. Or a glossy picture book from my shelves which is not often opened. We can find an inspiring world waiting for us within our own four walls.

Really, this is something that could be done a few times a week or even most days without any deleterious effects on our time and productivity. In fact, it could *help* with both.

When we feel refreshed and rejuvenated, we return to our tasks with a new focus. We gain fresh ideas and have a renewed sense of enthusiasm. We are rested and ready to tackle the remainder of our day!

And sometimes, just sometimes, small problems that were nagging us suddenly resolve. We think of an idea and it all works out. I truly believe these mini-miracles come from switching our mind to something else. Magical things can happen when you spend a little time in *your* contemplation corner.

30 Chic Days at Home inspired action:

Imagine the peacefulness of sitting in a five-star hotel contemplation corner and see how you could bring the same feeling into your home, even just for a little while. You are that wealthy lady sitting back with time to spare. You give yourself the time.

Find a space to set up. Set a tray with your drink, some reading material and maybe even a tiny dish of something delicious to nibble on. Make your tray pretty, with a cloth and even a bud vase. Serve it to yourself as if you were a five-star guest.

Day 13 -
Uplift yourself with happy journalling

It's fantastically enjoyable to be inspired by others and learn from their message. I do this a lot. I love reading books, listening to podcasts, watching YouTube videos, and studying the various courses I've purchased over the years.

And, it feels good when you balance your intake with your own creation by journalling, blogging, and writing inspiration for yourself: generally discovering what lights *you* up.

By doing this you can explore such concepts as:

- 'Happy lists' of what makes you feel happy, content and blessed at that particular time.
- 'Wouldn't it be amazing?' lists of your biggest dreams, hopes, and goals.

- 'Ideal self' visualisations in any area of your life that you desire to upgrade next, such as your wardrobe, health goals, or lifestyle wishes.
- Brainstorming loads of inspiring actions towards a specific outcome, such as 'How can I uplevel my personal style without spending any money?' or 'What are ten fun and easy ways in which I can improve my health?'

Creating your own bespoke inspiration doesn't have to be difficult, dry or require advanced level skills. You can make it as fancy or as simple as you want. I don't decorate my journals at all, as with bullet journalling or scrapbook type journalling. Yes I choose pretty notebooks, but then they're just filled with my lush and beautiful words. That's all. Each of us gets to choose the way in which we most enjoy inspiring ourselves.

You can also journal anywhere you like. On vacation, in the bath, on the bus going to work, on an aeroplane, with breakfast, cozy in bed, or waiting for an appointment. There are so many places to grab a quick little pocket of inspirational time!

And aside from writing in journals, you can also read them back for extra oomph. Maybe you want to borrow a bit of enthusiasm for a project or goal that you started working towards and then lost your way a little bit.

It's fun too, to see what you were thinking at a certain point in time. And it's *extra*-fun to see that an issue which was bothering you and you were working out what to do about it, has totally resolved. That's when you can see the magic of doing mindset work.

Or for something a little different, you can start a private or anonymous Blogger or Instagram account and create your dream fantasy life there. There is something fun about writing freely when no-one knows who you are. You may end up connecting with like-minded people over time as well.

30 Chic Days at Home inspired action:

You don't need special training or to read a book on journalling. Just find yourself a notebook or scrapbook, and plan to fill a page today. There is no timer to set and no word count. Just a page to fill out. Sometimes it's those last few lines that are the most challenging, but it feels good to complete a page. And date your pages too, that's always interesting!

If you feel that journalling has become a little stale for you or you have resistance towards it, start out with a fresh slate by starting a new social media or blog account. That way you can incorporate beautiful pictures from Pinterest along with your own words.

Choose a pretty name, like an alter ego, and dream up your most fabulous life and how you'd like to be. Follow accounts with the same goals. Tell no-one about this account, it's just for you to be your truly authentic self, since no-one you know is watching!

Day 14 -
Introduce pampering spa touches

As you create your ideal serene spa life, why not consider adding pampering touches to every corner of your home? There is no downside! And even the cost is minimal, because I imagine you'll have many of these items in your home already. And the rest, like my first point below, are *très* inexpensive.

There are endless ways you can add these cosseting details into your home; here are some of my favourites:

- Thick, soft tissues in just about every room.
- Hand cream in multiple places: the car, by the sofa, by your bed, on your office desk, in the bathroom, in your lady basket, and a tiny tube in your handbag. When it's there, you will put it

on. Massage it into your wrists, and push your cuticles back too.

- Saved-up hotel slippers for putting on after you've moisturized your feet with a luscious body cream before bed. Or fluffy house socks if you don't have spa slippers or want to walk around the house. These kinds of socks don't cost much, so buy yourself a few new pairs every year.
- A small, neat stack of glossy magazines for a quick browse.
- Using white towels. I went through a coloured towel phase but have recently started using white towels again. I love both, but the simplicity of only having white towels to wash is wonderful, and they look very 'spa luxe'!
- A cozy throw rug in the cooler season for wrapping up.
- Small bottles of sparkling water in the fridge.
- A bud vase with a few tiny fresh flowers in it, or a faux flower spray.

Even just reading through this list, don't you feel spoiled already? As with staying in a five-star hotel, or going for a treatment at a fancy spa, you feel cared for, as if your every wish was already there for you. It makes for such a nice atmosphere to be in an environment where those pampering touches are present, and you get to do it for yourself at home as well.

30 Chic Days at Home inspired action:

Choose a few favourites from this list and start dotting them around the house today. Put tissues on your shopping list. Dig out all those little tubes of gift hand creams and distribute them into different rooms where you sit. And actively look for ways in which you can pamper yourself. Make it a fun project to find them all out!

Day 15 -

Be in a soft, hushed atmosphere

I know for myself I can easily crash around putting things away (emptying the dishwasher!) and yelling at the dogs to 'be quiet!' when they go nuts barking at birds outside. You might be the same.

And, we can just as easily make life more tranquil and pleasant for ourselves by doing everything *as quietly as possible*. We can make our home a serene haven of calm for ourselves and our family.

We can:

- Put clean cups and plates away without clanking them.
- Shoosh the dogs in a calm manner.
- Walk to the room someone is in to talk to them rather than calling down the hall.
- Speak using our 'inside voice'.

- Think when to speak at all: is it necessary? Or are we just filling air?
- Move around the house in an intentionally calm and contented manner, quietly doing what we want to do.
- Keep the volume lower on our television if we are watching it, or turn it off if we aren't.
- Play music at a gentle level.

And at work too, we can be quietly productive, not bothering others with noise, loud sighs, and intrusive chatter. Is there anything worse than an annoyingly loud coworker? I think not!

But if you are at home by yourself mostly, as I am, you do it for yourself. It's lovely to feel settled and calm, and being intentionally quiet is one way you can do this for yourself.

When the house is peaceful my pet dogs seem calmer and quieter too. It makes sense. They pick up on my energy. You may find the same with children and other family members.

You get to set the tone for your home. It can be serene and harmonious, or loud and chaotic. You get to choose which you prefer. You don't need to boss anyone else, just lead by example. You don't even need to let anyone know what you're doing, just start being that way. Have some words as a sort of mantra to help you remember.

Imagine having 'gentle and calm' or 'peaceful

vibes' or 'my harmonious home' as a touchpoint to guide you. Write your phrase down on a sticky note, or type a note into your phone.

30 Chic Days at Home inspired action:

If this chapter appeals to you, decide now that you are going to become calmer, more centred, and that you want to develop a deep sense of inner peace. Let this desire settle within you, and carry on with your day from that place. Gather a few words to remind you, and repeat them to yourself often. Lessen the noise that is around you and be intentional about the kind of atmosphere you want for your home.

Day 16 -

Nourish yourself three times a day

If you were booked into a high-end spa, you can bet that your meals would be a symphony of fresh zingy tastes, and nutrient-dense too.

But how do we translate this into our own home, when the people we live with might prefer less healthy foods, and we have our favourites that we don't want to give up either. We want to be healthier, but we don't want to change anything!

What I have found helpful is to make tiny changes, and tweak different parts of my meals to increase the nutrient content and make them healthier. And, don't try to change everything at once. Choose one small thing and do that for a while. Then, when it's become a happy habit for you, add another in.

I did this for myself, and now that it's been many years since that decision to add fresh produce into my meals more, I can offer you a few examples.

You could:

- Eat an apple after lunch, even if lunch was fast food!
- Add a pre-made side salad to your dinner, regardless of what you are having.
- Slice fresh fruit to have with your breakfast.

The key with all of these kinds of ideas is to have 'the extra bit' (your new healthy addition) washed, sliced if needed, and ready to go when you serve yourself your meal.

Have an apple washed in your bag when you go through the drive-through. I don't eat fast food because I am celiac and nothing is ever gluten-free, but I am also realistic about what people eat! Wash, slice, and store fruit in a small GladWare container. Make your salad in portions too. That way, all you need to do is 'grab and go'. *Lessen the barrier between you and your healthy additions.*

I promise you will feel great with the added fresh nutrition. When I started having NutriBullet smoothies for breakfast, my cells would practically zing with happiness after I'd had one. I could feel it quite literally!

Mother Nature provides so much goodness for us, let's be grateful and nourish ourselves with her fresh produce!

30 Chic Days at Home inspired action:

Choose one meal to add a fresh component to, and start with that. My husband often takes dinner leftovers to work to heat up for lunch. In the past few months he started packing a small tub of celery sticks to add to his meal. He said they actually enhance the taste because they provide a refreshing thirst quench, and crunchiness too.

Day 17 -
Partake in boudoir time

If you have read any of my other books, you've likely heard me talk about 'boudoir time'. But I have to mention it here too, because regular boudoir time is probably one of the top ways I love to feel relaxed and peaceful, and it makes for a great night's sleep too.

Boudoir time is not what you might think... in my world it means going to our bedroom a little earlier than my husband (while he is still watching tv); basically retiring to your bedroom an hour or so earlier than you might normally. I don't do this every single night, just as and when I feel like it.

When you go, take some thoughtfully chosen reading material in your lady basket with you – a gently inspiring book, or an issue of your favourite 'ladylike' magazine (like *Victoria* is for me). You might even take your journal and pen for a little inspirational session. Make yourself an herbal tea too – preferably chamomile or a sleepy time tea blend.

While your tea is steeping, wash your face and apply a mask, and also moisturise your hands and feet with a rich, creamy lotion (put fluffy bed socks on your feet, they will feel wonderful).

Then, prop yourself up in bed with a couple of pillows behind your back and read for twenty minutes or so while your mask sets. Once this is done and you have finished your tea, wash your mask off with a clean face flannel and a basin of very-warm water. Apply your serum, eye cream and night cream – whatever you normally use.

From the mask's active ingredients and your gentle washing, your face will be plumped out, pink, soft, and happy. I always marvel at how smooth my skin is the morning after I've partaken in boudoir time!

For a little added extra relaxation, play soft background music too. When you combine all of these components leading up to bedtime, you will have a restful and restorative sleep. I know I always do.

30 Chic Days at Home inspired action:

Spend a few minutes designing your boudoir time. What time ideally would you start? How long would you like to relax for? What music will you play? Do you have a small Bluetooth speaker you could use? What will you read? Gather a few books, and buy yourself some bedtime tea if you don't already have a relaxing herbal tea. I hope you really enjoy your boudoir time tonight!

Day 18 -

Browse your style files

Do you have a stash of torn-out magazine pages in a folder? Articles printed out from websites? If you're like me, you collect these inspiring tidbits but often don't even remember they are there.

But when you do come across them again? You discover a wealth of inspiration, motivation, and encouragement. And the fun thing too, is that you will find a sense of cohesiveness that is very soothing. Simply by the act of collecting what has inspired you over time, you find out what is most important to you; what you value.

Maybe your 'style files' are full of fashion, home décor, gentle homemaking, and feminine self-development as mine are. Or perhaps yours comprise garden design notes, floral displays, and the beauty of nature. Or crafting ideas, knitting patterns, and things to make with your hands.

Sometimes you will have outgrown certain aspects of your style files, so it's good to have a prune out as you go too.

As you gather ways to find peace and relaxation in your daily life, consider that the act of perusing your style files is a very necessary part of this. Take five minutes to dip in, and see what inspired action comes of it.

Take this time as your personal retreat when you slow down and reimagine what is possible. You are that elegant lady gathering inspiration for her new season's wardrobe or garden, or finding fresh self-care ideas.

I always find myself relaxing effortlessly when I read through my collection of inspiring words and pictures. There is a sense of nostalgia as I remember what has inspired me previously.

I don't tear magazine pages out so much now, that has moved to Pinterest, so my magazine pages are a door to the past, sometimes as far back as the 1990s. When I decluttered my large magazine collection I went through a lot of the issues and kept the pages that spoke to me. It's so fun to have them all stored together.

I have printed out some of my favourite online articles to intersperse with the magazine pages, and I also have some hand-written pages where I have made notes of ideal ways I'd like to be, and followed prompts in books such as *Style Statement* (2008, Danielle LaPorte and Carrie McCarthy), and *Daring to Be Yourself* (1990, Alexandra Stoddard).

However your style files are organised (or disorganised!) I hope you have a pleasurable read, maybe during your boudoir time.

30 Chic Days at Home inspired action:

If you have also collected inspiration over the years, get them out one day and have a look through. Buy yourself some inexpensive display books to house them if you don't have an organisation system, and put them somewhere you will read them regularly.

Day 19 -
Indulge yourself every day

During a spa day, *everything* feels pampered - your face, your body, and your soul. Well, the soul pampering comes from the physical pampering. I've never done an actual full spa day, but I have had facials or massages. All these kinds of treatments feel delightfully restorative, but if you're a thrifty girl like me, sometimes the cost can take away from the pleasure. That's why I like to treat myself daily, at home.

It's *free* because you get to use the products you've bought or been given, and once you start telling yourself, 'Yes I do actually have the time', all these 'indulgences' become habits. At some stage you'll be happily surprised at just how much you do to spoil yourself. It's wonderful! And, your face, body and soul will be thanking you. You'll have softer skin, a more youthful appearance, and any underlying martyr feeling will be long gone, lost to the mists of time.

Daily indulgence starts at the beginning of the day for me. My shower is stocked with a small array of face and body products. I alternate between a foaming wash and an exfoliating wash on my face. And I always have a lovely soap. Plus I have shower gel to use on my long handled poufy brush to do my back. Everything in my shower I use at least once a week (such as my facial exfoliant or pumice stone for my heels), but mostly the items are used every day. I do *not* keep in my shower 'wish' products that I think I'll use but never do.

Then, when I'm finished in the shower and have dried off, I like to smother myself literally from top to toe in a deliciously scented rich body lotion. I change the brands and fragrances every time I buy a new one. It feels fresh and new to try different products.

Then I finish off with a body spray and some perfume. You won't find any fragrance-free products in my bathroom!

However you prefer *y*our products, use them daily and really pamper yourself. I promise you it doesn't take 'that' much longer than going without. And your skin will be soft and supple for life if you make moisturising a habit.

I hope I've convinced you to spend a little time on your legs and arms and everywhere else (bum cheeks, shoulders, decolletage, and stomach). Do it every day for a week and you will feel *transformed*.

30 Chic Days at Home inspired action:

Gather up all your lovely body products and commit to using them. They don't last forever, so start to enjoy them and pamper yourself at the same time. Be that wealthy lady of leisure as she indulges herself each morning, even if you know you will be heading off to work soon. What better way to start the day!

Day 20 -
Love herbal tea

Nothing says spa time like an herbal tea – hot or chilled. Maybe like me you 'love' herbal tea, but sometimes forget that, and it seems boring to you. Or maybe it's that you love the 'idea' of herbal tea. Then, when you make yourself a cup, you remember all over again how good it is!

I love fruit infusions, mint tea, chamomile, even green tea (but only with lemon or ginger).

There are many luxurious herbal teas around now. As part of a facial I had recently I was given a *très* fancy herbal tea in a takeaway cup. I looked up the brand and maybe I'll treat myself to a box one day (it's called Storm+India and the tea bags are handmade from fabric!) It was so, so delicious that I thought I might actually be able to justify the cost. I haven't yet, but you never know.

Thinking about it though, I'll spend money on

treat foods such as snacks, but I wouldn't on a healthy treat such as a high-end herbal tea? Something is a little wrong in my mind if I have no problem with one but not the other. It's something to think about as I continue to upgrade what I consume.

There are many bespoke brands around these days and they offer tea bags, as well as loose leaf tea in tins which can be more economical. If you have a teacup with a removeable strainer you're all set up!

And of course you could make fresh herb tea if you want to go one step further, because really, herb teas are just dried herbs. Imagine preparing your own tea with fresh herbs. That really is being extra. Fresh mint or other herbs are quick to steep in boiling water.

And, in the summer, making chilled herbal tea is wonderful. I soak my 'green tea with lemon' flavoured teabag in cold water for fifteen minutes and then remove it, and it is delicious in my drink bottle. With mint tea I leave the bag in and it's so refreshing. Especially if you make it the night before and store it in the fridge to properly chill, or add ice cubes if you forgot to do that.

Coffee or black tea with milk always seems more appealing when I forget how much I like herbal tea, but it really is an excellent addition to one's drinks regime. Zero calories, delicious taste, and probably even health benefits too. And, apart from green tea, there is no caffeine so you will be adding to, not detracting from, your hydration.

30 Chic Days at Home inspired action:

You don't have to give up your coffee in order to become an herbal tea lady. Simply choose one time each day when you will make yourself an herbal tea. Maybe after dinner for a relaxing bedtime drink. Or in a bottle to keep on your desk in the summer. Next time you're at the food store, look at the herbal tea selections and see if there is one you'd like to try. Or, if you already have some at home, commit to using it up before you buy any more.

Day 21 -
Take time to dream

What is that aspirational life you have always imagined yourself living? And how does it compare to how you live today? I always dreamed of a luxuriously creative life, and me with an elegant personal style. What about you? Were you going to be sporty and outgoing? Or work in high-end floral display? The art world?

Whatever your long-ago dreams were, see how you can infuse little details into your daily life today. Bring your desires back to life. Go to gallery openings. Watch a YouTube video on floral art and learn how to do the arrangements yourself. Put together a stylish outfit from your closet and include a scarf or costume jewellery for a little flair.

For me, I've been enjoying my sewing machine more, making home décor pieces and upcycling saved denim. I've been journaling, and making my home my own work of art by streamlining, organising and pottering around. I'm a happy homebody, but maybe you are someone who wants to get out more, travel more.

Remember your dreams for yourself. It will feel so good to give that girl inside of you air. She will take you by the hand and lead you forward, introducing petite and artful modifications to elevate your days.

Take the time to visualise how your life would be if *everything* was perfect. Brian Tracy calls it 'The Magic Wand Technique'. He says to write down what your life would be like if you could wave a magic wand and have everything become exactly as you want it. How would you look? How do you dress? Where do you live? Who do you live with? What's in your kitchen? How much money do you have?

I like to use this as a meditation before I fall asleep at night, imagining my perfect life in exquisite detail. As you lie back comfortably, consider your desires. Write them down the next day and act on them in any way you can. Mine don't cost a lot of money, but they do require intention, effort, and disregarding what others might think of me.

But it's worth it, don't you think? To truly live as you have always imagined? And it can be done. You can decide to be the one who is steering your ship, rather than a passenger sitting on it simply floating with the current. You can be your own captain – hop up there into the driver's seat!

30 Chic Days at Home inspired action:

Remember what you have enjoyed doing in the past. Why did you stop? Is there something creative or fun that you can pick up again? Table tennis? Knitting? Jogging? These are all things I've enjoyed previously that appeal now. What about you?

Day 22 -
Decrease your to-do list

Life is busy for many of us. No matter how calm and serene we'd like our days to be, it somehow never works out like that don't you find? Days go by in a flash. And there always seems to be something we have to deal with outside of our normal routine.

I don't have children, but I am at a stage in life where there are aging parents, and other older family members who require care from me as well. And it's at times like this that your free time can shrink down to nothing. Chores are put off, and your only respite is five minutes of reading before bed.

But even in normal times when there are no pressing issues, it feels like I have a lot to do. You may feel the same.

But no-one is a superwoman no matter how charmed and easy their life may seem from the outside. We all deal with our own life situations, and also want to keep mentally healthy as well.

That's why it is so important not to be bogged down by your to-do list. To not feel like a failure at life if you don't do everything perfectly. Spoiler alert: no one does! Everyone is struggling in their own way. This is what I have found out from chatting with others. We all feel like we should be doing better. Well I'm here to say *Let's kick this corrosive guilt out the door*. It has no place in our life!

Mostly I am an upbeat person, but I do have my days where it is impossible to gain traction. Thankfully these days are not too frequent, but I do have to constantly monitor myself and also be kind with my self-talk. I don't know if it's common, or, as I suspect, something to do with being an introvert or even part of having a creative mind. But I do know that I can easily become burnt out if I don't sometimes let things slide.

If this sounds like you, pare back your high standards when you need to. Relax your shoulders. See what really needs to be done, and forget the rest. Until tomorrow at least. And, if you can do a job quickly and imperfectly, do that rather than having it hanging over you for another day.

Keep your life as simple as you can. Aim for a settled, calm existence and remember this when you are tempted to take on something extra. And... breathe out.

30 Chic Days at Home inspired action:

Give yourself a pass, starting today. Look at your schedule with fresh eyes and remember that yes you are an integral part in other peoples lives, but you are also here on this earth to enjoy a pleasurable existence, not just to be the chief tidier and cook. Remove non-essential jobs from your already burdened shoulders. Dole out a few jobs to others. Find space to relax. And don't feel bad about it!

Day 23 -
Be slow

Today I invite you to slow everything down. And I mean *everything*. Slow down how you move, how you think, how you walk, and how you talk. Even if it seems almost painful to go so slow, do it.

Try it for even one day; you can put a sticky note up in front of your computer screen or wherever you will see it most – 'S L O W'.

Slowing down enables you to have space to think, process, and be present. And more than that, it just feels amazing. Let your body relax, soften, and be at peace. You will still get just as much done; it's quite incredible. And maybe you will realise just how much you have been rush, rush, rushing all day every day. No wonder you can't sleep at night!

If you don't believe me, try it. You might forget, and that's okay. Just get back into slow when you remember. You'll need a few reminders since you've been going so fast for so long. When you remind yourself to be slow today it feels *so good*. Like a massage for your insides.

There are so many benefits to slowing down.

- You restore your balance and equilibrium and generally feel better in yourself.
- You make better decisions because you are not in a rush, and can receive all the information you need.
- You are more productive and have more energy.
- You can connect with others easier and actually have a useful conversation with them.
- Your stress levels will drop and burnout will not be looming up in front of you.

If you are someone who always feels in a rush and as if you are behind (like me!), you are in for a treat.

And if the word slow doesn't resonate with you, try *measured*, *intentional*, *consistent*, or *systematic*. Imagine having a day where you focus on being *intentional* with every thought, step, and action. Or you decide to be *measured* in how you approach your day. It would be quite calming and restorative!

30 Chic Days at Home inspired action:

Accept this invitation to slow down and see how that would look in your own life. But first of all, slow your physical body. Breathe deeply in a calm manner. Be more measured in your movements. Do one thing at a time. Tidy things away as you go. When you notice something is out of place, address it. Be a sweeping presence in your home, creating peace wherever you go. And enjoy the tranquilness that comes with intentional movement!

Day 24 -
Create a sense of calm in your home

Following on from slowing down how you do things, so too could you think about how to make your home feel calmer and more peaceful. Wouldn't that be wonderful? Imagine walking in the door after work to *your restful haven.*

How can we do this though? When we've had a long day and just want to crash? Here are a few of my favourite tips:

- **Prep your evening dinner** the night before or even that morning. Vegetables are washed and sliced in the fridge. Your protein of choice is flavoured, chopped and ready to cook – or perhaps it's cooked already and just needs adding to your meal.

- **Have less to look after** in your home. Clear

cluttery corners or spaces. Spend fifteen minutes a day doing one small space. Be a little ruthless getting rid of things that you know you will never use but keep 'just in case'. You will feel so light when you bin or donate those things.

- **Clean dust away** with microfibre cloths and have a small basket in the laundry to drop them in afterwards. I have a stash of clean cloths that are easy to grab, and I do a hot wash once a month. You often don't need a cleaning product; maybe dampen the cloth slightly, but even a dry cloth collects the dust and keeps your home feeling nice with minimal effort.

- **Keep on top of jobs** such as laundry. Many people do one load a day and I find this works for me too. Whichever basket is the fullest, I do that one. And one load a day never gets overwhelming. Do other tasks quickly and don't worry if they are not one hundred percent perfect.

- **Create lovely touches** in your home such as a candle burning on the sideboard or coffee table, a few recent magazines stacked, or a good book inviting you to sit and read. Even if you don't have time to read right now, just the suggestion relaxes you. I like to place pretty cloth coasters on side tables for a hot drink, and have music playing too. Imagine you work in a five-star hotel and you want to have things be extra nice for your guests. Do this for yourself and your own family.

These are just a few of my favourite ways. I hope they spark of some of your own for you!

30 Chic Days at Home inspired action:

In your journal, ask yourself 'How can I make my home feel calmer and more peaceful?' and start writing down ideas specific to *your* home. There will be spots that bother you, so write those down and you might get easy ideas on how to fix them. Walk around your home as a guest and see what stands out. Take at least one small action today to increase the sense of calm in your home. Yes it's another job to do, but I find that they don't take long to do and they actually make me feel happier afterwards. And more energised as well!

Day 25 -
Always be streamlining

Most people bring new items into their home just about every time they leave the house. I know this is true for me. I'm either going to buy everyday necessities such as food or toiletries, or less frequent purchases such as new clothes, bedding, furniture, crafting supplies, books, or home décor. It is effortless to fill our home up, but a lot more hassle to empty it out, which is why so many of us end up with a cluttered space!

One solution is to make the 'emptying out' as much a routine as your regular grocery shop. Every week look around at what you are not using that can be donated, declutter clothes that you no longer like (or fit), and throw away broken items if they cannot be mended. Use up food items in your kitchen as ingredients in a meal instead of buying everything new each week.

After you start doing this, you will notice how much 'quieter' your home feels, simply because there is less stuff in it.

And if you get stuck on items that might have cost you a bit of money and you are holding them back to sell online to try and recoup some of your costs, consider this advice from Peter Walsh.

He says instead of looking at the money you've spent and how you can get it back, decide to donate these items to your favourite charity and reframe it for yourself. Rather than say, 'look at how much money all this stuff is worth, you spent it and now you wasted it', say 'look how much you are benefiting this charity with your donations'. You could even go one step further and estimate for yourself how much those items might raise for 'your' charity.

This mindset shift helped me donate a handful of items that I had been holding onto because I wanted to sell them online but hadn't yet because of all the bother, and I didn't really fancy strangers turning up to my house to collect the bigger items either. After hearing Peter's advice I took everything to our local SPCA thrift store as a donation to the pets.

The items were in excellent as-new condition and I knew they might fetch a few hundred dollars in total. It's not that I wouldn't go out of my way for $200, but it felt *so good* to let it all go in an instant and have the space in my home and my mind. I actually felt richer as a result even though I didn't receive any money. Truly!

Now I know everyone is at different financial places in their life, and when I was younger I did sell things online and get $20 or $40 for them. It helped us out when we were saving for our first home and then making headway into our mortgage.

But now I am in my fifties and our thriftiness is finally paying off it feels really good for me to 'pay it forward' to the SPCA for all the good work they do, and donate those slightly better items.

30 Chic Days at Home inspired action:

Make streamlining and decluttering a regular part of your routine. Spend fifteen minutes a day tidying a hotspot and see if there is anything you can get rid of.

And, if you can, consider donating items that you might have deemed 'too good' or 'too expensive' to a charity that is close to your heart, if you too have a pile that never seems to make it online to sell!

Day 26 -
Practice reflexology daily

Something relaxing you can do for yourself at virtually zero cost and which only takes minutes of your time, is to massage your own feet. I can almost guarantee you already have a pot of cream or body butter that you don't often use. Get it out, and put it on your nightstand.

And tonight, before you hop into bed, massage each foot with this cream. I like to keep a pair of hotel slippers by my bed so that I don't put my creamy feet on the carpet. You can also use a pair of fluffy bed socks as an alternative. I cannot tell you how good it feels to do a two-minute self-massage on each foot and then put fluffy socks on. Your feet will be floating!

I do the same when I change into my loungewear at the end of the day. I like to wear soft socks around the house, so when I change, I massage body butter into my feet then too. I really don't think you can do it too often! And once you start doing it, you will become hooked and it will turn into a wonderful habit.

If you do this, combined with keeping a pumice stone in your shower and using it on the heels and soles of your feet a few times a week, you will probably never need an expensive pedicure. When I go to get my toes done in the summer, my lady tells me that my heels are in perfect shape and she really can't make them any better! And it all comes from daily care.

There is another fabulous benefit when you massage your own feet each day, and that is the benefits of reflexology. According to Egyptian history dating back thousands of years, our feet (and hands) have pressure points that relate to all the different parts of our body.

I haven't studied reflexology enough to know if all this is true, but I do know that I feel rejuvenated after a professional foot massage, and also how good my feet feel as I fall asleep at night after pampering them with my own self-massage.

30 Chic Days at Home inspired action:

You know you already have a rich body cream in your cupboard. Go and get it out and start using it tonight, or even now. Show your feet love and attention; they will be so happy to receive it. When you think about it, they are the most hard-working and probably most forgotten part of our body.

As you massage, pretend you know what you are doing and focus on different parts of your sole. Notice where you have tender spots and focus there gently. And if you're extra inspired, search out a 'map' of your feet online and see what those tender spots represent. Just search for 'reflexology map' or 'foot map'.

Day 27 -

Find five minutes for stretching

Stretching and yoga are those things that feel amazing when you do them, but do you find that you often forget? You forget to stretch, and you forget that you want to 'do yoga' for your posture and peace of mind. Me too!

And, it's just as easy to stand up right now and stretch your arms high above your head. To feel straight and tall and take a few deep breaths. To arch backwards slightly and look up. And to do shoulder rolls when you lower your arms down.

Imagine making it a practice to do even these simple stretches five times a day. Some things are so small that we think they can't make a difference to how we feel and how healthy and limber our body is, but everything counts. It all counts. No movement, or change in our diet is too small to be worth the effort.

So please join me in this mini-mission to pamper ourselves with luxurious stretching. Set your alarm for five different times to remind you if you want to. Personally alarms like this annoy me, so I'd rather write a sticky note that prompts me each time I see it. Imagine seeing 'Stretch your beautiful body!' as a reminder. What a wonderful invitation.

And then, you might even do a few yoga moves such as standing with your feet astride and reaching over one side of your head with your arm outstretched reaching tall, and then the other way. There are simple yoga stretches you can search for online if you need inspiration.

But like most good things in life, all it will cost you is a few minutes of your time and a little effort. And the payoff is immense! Imagine getting into a habit of stretching every hour. You'd stand up from your desk, or the sofa, and have a fabulously languid stretch. If you feel self-conscious, go into a room where no-one else is.

If it's at home I'm sure you won't mind if your family sees you, but at work you might want to go into the kitchen or bathroom. But maybe if others see you standing up and stretching by your computer, they will feel like they can as well. Don't wait until your back is cricked and you feel like an L-shape from sitting for so long. But if this is where you are starting from, that's okay too.

30 Chic Days at Home inspired action:

Find a way to remind yourself to stretch that works well for you. Word it in an appealing way so that you *want* to stretch, not feel obligated to. Search online for 'simple back stretches' or 'desk stretches' to give you some ideas. You can even stretch sitting down. Enjoy your luxurious stretching!

Day 28 -
Connect with girlfriends

I love being a happy homebody and spending time by myself. It's how I recharge, and if you are a homebody too you might feel the same. But it's also wonderful to share our peaceful home with others. I love to entertain at home because it's a nice place to be, and it is usually more relaxing – not to mention less expensive – than going out.

It's great to do things as a couple, but I especially love spending time with other ladies for a change. My two favourite ways to do this at home are:

Hosting afternoon tea. I mostly do this for family: aunties and cousins. There is usually half-a-dozen of us and everyone brings a plate, not because I ask them to, but just because they do. I like to make something sweet and something savoury. Whenever I make egg finger sandwiches with the crusts cut off they are all eaten! Or savoury eggs for a non-gluten alternative. And some kind of cake or slice too. I don't often bake just for myself so it's a nice treat to make something yummy.

And my other favourite way is to **invite a girlfriend around for cheese and wine** and a little catchup. I always make sure to have dinner prepped and in the slow-cooker when I do this, as a 4pm start time can extend into dinner time!

Another thing I love about having people around at any time, is that it's a great motivator to have my house looking extra clean, tidy, and lovely. I light candles, choose a playlist, and add all those extra touches such as a few roses from the garden in a bud vase, or compiling a new ornamental display on our sideboard. It's just as nice for me as it is for my guests, and the next day I get to enjoy the benefits of my tidy, pretty home.

Sometimes we realise we haven't hosted anyone in a while just because it hasn't occurred to us. This thought came to me last week, so I emailed a lovely neighbour, and we are having a wine together at my place this afternoon. It's going to be so nice to see her.

30 Chic Days at Home inspired action:

Even if you think your place is 'too small' or 'too cluttered' to have anyone over, book something in. If it's for a week or two's time, you now have an enticing deadline to tidy up your space. For some of us an impending visitor is the best motivation!

You can put together a simple menu (mine tonight is two types of cheese, two types of crackers, and red grapes, so simple!) and enjoy this time catching up with your friends.

Day 29 -

Develop morning and evening rituals

There has been a lot written about morning routines, and the less talked-about nighttime routines, but I propose that we call them morning and evening *rituals* instead. Doesn't this sound more calming? And less routine?

Even for people who don't write for a living like I do, words hold a lot of weight. They can reframe how we think about something and all for changing a few letters. A ritual to me seems sacred, whereas a routine sounds a little... dull. Rituals sound like our best and most favourite things, while routine has a touch of the *shoulds* about it. In fact, I like to exchange the word routine for regime. If it's something I want to include in my day, I create a *regime*. It just sounds more chic!

No matter what you call it, whether you prefer a regime or a ritual, or even a plain old routine, there is a gentle sense of measuredness when you have a set of actions morning and night that work for you.

To get your own thinking started, please let me share my favourite morning and evening rituals. I have built these up over the years and it's wonderful to have things to look forward to as the bookends of my day.

Morning

- Rising early and writing my books with hot tea.
- Going for a walk on my treadmill while I watch something enjoyable such as a fun movie or an inspiring YouTube video.
- Walking the dogs down the road or in our paddock.
- Making a green smoothie packed full of goodness for breakfast.
- Having a long shower and pampering my body with sweet-smelling products.

Evening

- Doing a Pilates class on YouTube in the late afternoon (this is a habit in progress).
- Prepping dinner well before dinnertime (not right when I'm about to start cooking).
- Playing a walking tour on YouTube on our television, with appropriate music while my husband Paul and I chat after work.
- Enjoying a glass of wine with dinner (we have a regime where we each have a glass, and the

other half of the bottle is sealed for the next night).

- Doing a five-minute tidy of the kitchen and living area (the dishes have already been done, but putting items away such as remote controls in the basket under our coffee table makes for a pleasing vista in the morning).
- Cleansing my skin before bed in a leisurely manner and applying night cream.
- Going to bed early with a novel and reading for half an hour.

I love my morning and evening rituals so much. And they aren't set in stone either, although I have been doing them for many years, decades even. But there is something freeing about being able to change things up if I want to.

I tried for years to implement a yoga practice and it hung over me like a dark cloud because I never did. Then one day I decided to try Pilates and it was a revelation. It took a little while to get the habit in place but now I look forward to my late afternoon Pilates 'class' (I follow 'Move With Nicole' on YouTube).

No-one wants to feel trapped or like they 'should' do something, so give yourself the freedom to *only* do what feels good. When you do this you will find that ideas come naturally to you and you will be drawn to them. No effort required!

30 Chic Days at Home inspired action:

There might be things you do that you didn't even consider were a daily ritual, but when you write them down you can see that they are enjoyable, and you benefit from them. List your favourite things to do at each end of the day and see how you have started building your rituals already. Then add in things you'd love to do. Choose one to start with and once that is habitual, add another.

Look upon your daily rituals as things you do that strengthen you (in all ways, not just physically), nourish you, and provide pleasure, whether that is during or after. For example, it's not like I jump for joy at prepping my vegetables in the morning or at lunchtime, but when I come to cook that night and my fridge contains a bowl of washed, chopped vegetables, I am very happy to have them already done!

Day 30 -

Create your own spa day

What would you love to do if you had a completely free day with no work, jobs, or errands to do, and no-one to consider but yourself? Imagine creating the perfect 'spa day' for yourself, even if only on paper for now. And who knows, one day you might even have the guts to do it! A spa day is sort of like a 'duvet day' but more chic.

If it was me, I'd be at home, because that's my favourite place to be. I'd be by myself, as much as I love my family and friends. But I know I'd be meeting them for dinner later on. This would be the perfect mix of alone time and connectedness for my sensibility.

I'd start my day quite early, since I'm a lark, with a cup of tea and a little contemplation time. I'd prop myself up in bed with my journal and pen, and maybe a few books too. Then I would do some light exercise before my wholesome breakfast, and look forward to a wonderful day ahead. I'd do some sewing or other creative handwork, break for lunch, and spend the afternoon reading. I'd take the time to go for a stroll outside and enjoy the sun. Later in the day I'd do some stretches and tidy my space, ready for a relaxing evening with my loved one(s).

Just writing this out feels so restorative, and I haven't even done anything different, just dreamed on paper for five minutes. I might create a different day too, one where I do a little window shopping and research the upcoming season's fashions so I can redesign my seasonal wardrobe.

I think the most important time for any of us when we are designing our own perfect spa day is that we have free rein. Freedom of time, and only ourselves to please.

What would a lovely spa day look like for you? Would you sunbathe outside reading a book? Potter in the garden for pleasure? Have a craftathon? A pampering session in your bathroom using all your pretty products? Or maybe you'd check into an actual day spa for a treatment or two.

There are limitless ways in which we can spend our precious free time, but if you're anything like me, you somehow push those activities to the backburner. You feel guilty if you're 'doing nothing'.

But what if it was necessary for you to have these downtime activities? If a doctor prescribed them to you for your own wellbeing? That would make for an excellent prescription I think. Better than any pills!

Let's all try it. Let's design our own spa day and then, *do it*. It will be blocked out on our calendar. If we have to leave the house, so be it. Just say you have something very important to sort out. And then go. I know not many of us are likely to do this, even if it's a fun thought.

But please consider this final chapter a reminder that you get to relax too. You are not just the boss of the home who gets to pick up the slack in all areas. Your pleasure and enjoyment in life matters as much as anyone else's.

So take this chapter seriously and dream up all the ways in which you could fill a spa day, and then do it for real!

30 Chic Days at Home inspired action:

Design a couple of spa days – one at home and one out. List all the details that would make them fabulous, regardless of cost. Maybe your 'out' day has a helicopter ride! Or more realistically, perhaps seeing a movie by yourself and a cocktail afterwards, looking mysterious reading your book at the table.

And even if you don't do everything on your 'ideal spa day' list, at least you've had fun compiling it. And who knows, the mind works in mysterious ways, so maybe you'll conjure up something just from putting it out there. Have fun!

I sincerely hope you have enjoyed this little book, and that you've gained inspiration and found a few new ideas to live a more beautiful and serene life. It really is the simple touches that can add so much to our home life.

When I watch home makeover programmes on television it's always heartwarming to see how a simple declutter, deep clean and maybe a few light renovations can have such a profound effect on people.

And we can do this for ourselves when we focus on making our home feel more peaceful and relaxing. We don't have to have the television crew come in and expose our home to the world. We can be private and do it over time to suit our personality and our budget. We can make small changes that feel great to us.

Before I go, I'd love to leave you with twenty-one extra ways in which your home can become a calm haven for you and your family. These are tiny little touches that your family might not even notice you doing, but that will make a big difference to how good everyone feels.

So thank you for reading and please enjoy this final chapter!

21 *Ways to make your home a calm haven*

1. **Be intentional with the energy** you have in your home. Think 'calm', 'peaceful', and 'serene' or choose similar words that soothe you. Write them down if you want, and actively cultivate the feeling of these words with how you are.

2. **Lessen visual clutter** by putting things away as much as possible. If you don't use something often, find a spot for it in a cabinet. And if there is no room in the cabinet, see what else is in there. Do you remember the last time you used these things? Can you live without them?

3. **Simplify your décor colour scheme**. You don't have to go all-white, but there is something wonderful about choosing a few colours that you love and using them

throughout your home. Surround yourself with your favourites and you can't go wrong.

4. **Consider your home to be the most important place** for you and your family to recharge. You are the thermostat of your home, and how you treat it is what will filter through to others. When you start to view your home space as sacred, everyone else will pick up on that as well.

5. **Make it your mission to use up consumables** and not overstock. It's good to save money in sales, but very often we end up stockpiling items and then not using them and they become more of a burden than a blessing. I speak from experience! There will always be special offers on. Enjoy what you have, and also enjoy the good feeling that comes from buying an item *because you've actually run out of it*.

6. **Wear socks or bare feet inside**. Something that will make you feel calm and intentional, is to walk around *feeling* the ground. It feels very 'spa-like' for your toes to be able to move freely and for your feet to move in their natural way. In the summer I have bare feet inside, with my brightly coloured pretty toenails, and in the winter I buy myself a few new pairs of thick, cozy socks to wear around the house.

7. **Add a touch of green 'your way'**. I love the look of plants but do not enjoy the admin. So I have a few faux plants in my house. I live in the country and open my windows for fresh air most days, so I figure I can get away without having a Peace Lily! I know some people love tending to their plants but mine just stress me out. If you are the same, find yourself a good quality faux plant and enjoy the serenity of no-maintenance apart from a light dusting every once in a while.

8. **Filter the light that comes into a room by hanging sheer curtains**; especially if the view isn't that great or you need the privacy. But even if you don't, there is something very relaxing about having light-coloured sheers to soften and diffuse the light. You feel cosseted and enveloped by them.

9. **Be very, very clean**. One of my dear friends keeps an extremely clean home, and when I visit her it always feels peaceful and airy. And of course when you clean, you don't want clutter to move around, so regular cleaning leads to less 'stuff', which also leads to a soothing calmness.

10. **Curate your favourite books**. To make your home a haven of encouragement and inspiration, display your books and flick through them often. If you have so many that they are double stacked or packed in boxes, go

through them and donate those that no longer resonate with you. I have regular clear-outs – about once a year at a guess – because I buy books here and there and they do build up. When my shelves in the hall get too full it's time for another sort through! These hall shelves are the only place I keep books, so the space sets the limit for me.

11. **Identify a specific use for each room**. Your home will feel more like a tranquil retreat if your children's toys are in their room, and your work-from-home desk is tidy and tucked away. Look at your master bedroom and see if it reflects self-care and soul nourishment for you and your husband. If not, work out why and rectify the discrepancies as much as possible.

12. **Choose comforting textures**. Soft cottons in the summer, cozy rugs in the winter; however much you like to decorate for the seasons, choose textures that are pleasing to your touch. If any aren't, donate or bin them depending on their condition. Animal shelters always welcome old towels and blankets.

13. **Throw out or recycle anything that is not fixable**. Something that is guaranteed to needle away at me are broken or damaged items. I fix or have them fixed if I can, and if I can't I remove them immediately. An expensive glass with a

chip in the rim? Out. A favourite pair of good quality shoes that could be revitalised with new soles? They go into the car to be dropped off at the cobbler.

14. **Surround yourself with what you love**. It doesn't matter if your décor is against current trends. What matters is that it makes you happy. Own it, and love it.

15. **Limit sensory overload**. Some of us are more sensitive to sensory input than others, but I think everyone is affected to some degree. Loud noise, a lot of visual stimulation, clutter, overly full rooms; even just writing this is jarring me! So set out doing one room at a time, and limiting the 'noise', whether it is visual or auditory.

16. **Read from paper**. Even though I love my Kindle, I notice I am more present when I read from an actual book. I am also less distracted and unlikely to 'just look something up' if I leave my phone and tablet in my office, and read my book in the living room. Whenever you want a calmer ambience, put all your devices away in another room and you won't even notice they are gone.

17. **Think 'wellbeing'** when you are looking around your home, and ask yourself how you can infuse a sense of wellbeing into each room.

Can you make a cozy corner for yourself somewhere? Is your kitchen stocked with healthy foods? Is your bedroom tidy and ready for a restful sleep?

18. **Clear out hidden places**. Your home may seem like a peaceful space to guests, but you really know what is stuffed in drawers and closets, and it weighs heavily on you! I started going through a few areas that were quietly there in the background nagging at me. The most recent was my candle cupboard. I have been very good at using the scented candles I have before buying more, but my candle holder collection was too much. So I went through them all and kept only my very, very favourites. I donated around half of the total number I had, and now my candle cupboard is a pleasure to 'shop' from because I love everything in there!

19. **Reimagine rooms**. If you have the space, see if you can move items. Our living and dining areas are in the same room, and can be swapped around. It feels like a new room when I do this every year or so, just whenever I get into the mood, and it's also a good chance to deep clean as I move things. There is such a sense of elegant calm after doing something like this.

20. **Have a place for everything**. This is such a basic old-fashioned piece of advice, but worth

being reminded of. When an item has its own home, it is easy to put away and your place is kept tidier without effort. A sense of peace is promoted because you know where everything goes. If you have possessions that just seem to float around, never really belonging anywhere, find them a home. Or, donate if you think the real reason they float is because no-one ever uses them and won't miss them.

21. **Create family occasions**. Invite family members around on birthdays or special holidays. Stack a few board games and a pack of cards under your coffee table. Some of my happiest family memories have been hosting casual dinners in honour of someone. I've always found it best to invite first, and worry about the details later! They always work out, and even if I found it a bit stressful beforehand, I was always glad I'd done it afterwards.

To finish

Thank you for reading *30 Chic Days at Home Vol. 2: Creating a serene spa-like ambience in your home for soothing peace and relaxation*.

I do so hope you have enjoyed this book and that you gained a few new snippets of inspiration. If you have, I'd be grateful if you would consider placing a review on Amazon. It only takes five minutes – you don't need to write a lot, or even anything if you don't want to, you can just rate the book – and it means a lot to me as an author.

As well, it helps other lovely ladies find my work, and that is important to me because I think there is a dearth of feel-good inspiration in this world, particularly at the moment. And you know as well as I do that when you find something that makes you feel hopeful, inspired, and creative that that good feeling spreads like a carpet of wildflowers over time.

Please help me plant a few more seeds!

I wish you all the best, and I'll see you in my next book.

Fiona

About the author

Fiona Ferris is passionate about the topic of living well, in particular that a simple and beautiful life can be achieved without spending a lot of money.

Her books are published in five languages currently: English, Spanish, Russian, Lithuanian and Vietnamese. She also runs an online home study program for aspiring non-fiction authors.

Fiona lives in the beautiful and sunny wine region of Hawke's Bay, New Zealand, with her husband, Paul, their rescue cat Nina, rescue dogs Daphne and Chloe, and their cousin Micky dog.

To learn more about Fiona, you can connect with her at:
howtobechic.com
fionaferris.com
facebook.com/fionaferrisauthor
twitter.com/fiona_ferris
instagram.com/fionaferrisnz
youtube.com/fionaferris

Fiona's other books are listed on the next page, and you can also find them at:
amazon.com/author/fionaferris

Other books by Fiona Ferris

Thirty Chic Days: *Practical inspiration for a beautiful life*

Thirty More Chic Days: *Creating an inspired mindset for a magical life*

Thirty Chic Days Vol. 3: *Nurturing a happy relationship, staying youthful, being your best self, and having a ton of fun at the same time*

Thirty Slim Days: *Create your slender and healthy life in a fun and enjoyable way*

Financially Chic: *Live a luxurious life on a budget, learn to love managing money, and grow your wealth*

How to be Chic in the Winter: *Living slim, happy and stylish during the cold season*

How to be Chic in the Summer: *Living well, keeping your cool and dressing stylishly when it's warm outside*

A Chic and Simple Christmas: *Celebrate the holiday season with ease and grace*

The Original 30 Chic Days Blog Series: *Be inspired by the online series that started it all*

30 Chic Days at Home: *Self-care tips for when you have to stay at home, or any other time when life is challenging*

The Chic Author: *Create your dream career and lifestyle, writing and self-publishing non-fiction books*

The Chic Closet*: Inspired ideas to develop your personal style, fall in love with your wardrobe, and bring back the joy in dressing yourself*

The Peaceful Life*: Slowing down, choosing happiness, nurturing your feminine self, and finding sanctuary in your home*

Loving Your Epic Small Life*: Thriving in your own style, being happy at home, and the art of exquisite self-care*

The Glam Life*: Uplevel everything in a fun way using glamour as your filter to the world*

100 Ways *to Live a Luxurious Life on a Budget*

100 Ways *to Declutter Your Home*

100 Ways *to Live a European Inspired Life*

100 Ways *to Enjoy Self-Care for Gentle Wellbeing and a Healthy Body Image*

100 Ways *to be That Girl*

Printed in Great Britain
by Amazon

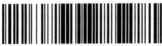

31767305R00065